The Autoimmune Paleo Cookbook: Manage Chronic Illness with Quick, Easy, and Flavorful Recipes

Disclaimer and Terms of Use: Effort has been made to ensure that the information in this book is accurate and complete, however, the author and the publisher do not warrant the accuracy of the information, text and graphics contained within the book due to the rapidly changing nature of science, research, known and unknown facts and internet. The Author and the publisher do not hold any responsibility for errors, omissions or contrary interpretation of the subject matter herein. This book is presented solely for motivational and informational purposes only.

Table of Contents

Beef Slow Cooker Recipes

Pot Roast with Gravy

Ingredients:

- 3 lbs. chuck roast
- 1 chopped onion
- 4 carrots, chopped
- Sliced 2 celery stalks
- 4 t Minced garlic
- 1 bay leaf
- Rosemary branches
- ¼ C broth
- Salt and pepper to taste

Direction:

I.   Add all of your vegetables and seasoning to slow cooker
II.   Add about ¼ of your broth to slow cooker, and season your roast
III.   Cover and cook for 6-8 hours on low
IV.   Use the juices in the slow cooker when done, you can add more bay leaf or rosemary if you would like

Brisket

Ingredients:
- 1 ½ lbs. brisket
- 3 C chicken stock
- 1 chopped onion
- 8 T minced garlic
- ½ can sliced mushroom
- ½ C sliced carrots
- 1 T garlic powder
- 1 T onion powder
- ½ tsp salt

Directions:

I.   Add stock, and seasoning with veggies into your slow cooker,

II. Add meat after seasoning with garlic powder, onion powder, and salt

III. Cook in slow cooker for 12-24 hours, checking on frequently

Bacon Cabbage Stew

Ingredients:

- ½ lbs. bacon, strips
- 3 lbs. chuck roast
- 2 red onions, chopped
- 1 T minced garlic
- 1 cabbage, chopped
- Salt and pepper to taste
- Organic thyme
- 1 C beef broth

Directions:

I.   Add everything in order as mentioned in ingredients list
II.   Cook on low for 7-8 hours
III. Serve

Veal Soup

Ingredients:

- 1-3 lbs. veal, chopped
- 2 sweet potatoes, cubed
- 2 sliced carrots
- 1 onion, sliced
- 6 T minced garlic
- Salt and pepper to taste
- ¼ tsp rosemary
- ¼ tsp savory
- ½ tsp thyme
- ¼ tsp basil
- ¼ tsp marjoram
- Parsley
- 1/8 tsp. oregano
- 1/8 tsp. tarragon
- 6 C beef broth

Directions:

I.   Add everything into your slow cooker, and let cook for 8 hours on low

II. Remove bones if any are present (some are deboned)

Cinnamon Roast and Onions

Ingredients:
- 3-4 lbs. chuck roast
- 2 onions, chopped
- 1-2 T cinnamon
- 2 T minced garlic
- Salt to taste

Directions:

I.   Add your onions first, into your slow cooker
II.   Season your roast well with all above seasonings
III.   Add roast, and broth and water
IV.   Let cook for 8 hours on low

Short Ribs

Ingredients:
- 4-5 lbs. beef short ribs

Asian Sauce

- ½ C coconut aminos
- ½ C broth
- 2 T apple cider vinegar
- 4 T honey
- 1 T grated ginger
- 5-6 T minced Garlic
- 1 T sesame oil
- Green onions

Directions:

I.   Add short ribs to your slow cooker
II.   Add all of your sauce ingredients, and stir well
III.   Toss sauce with ribs and cook on low for around 6-7 hours
IV.   Remove ribs after fully cooking and set aside to let cool
V.   Take the excess liquid from slow cooker and add it to a saucepan, and bring to a boil, then you want to let this simmer for about 10 minutes
VI.   Remove sauce from heat and add in the sesame oil and stir
VII.   Remove rib met from the bones and shred, using your fingers is always best
VIII. Add sauce over shredded ribs and enjoy

Nomads Chili

Ingredients:
- 2 chopped onions
- 4 T Minced garlic
- 2 lbs. ground beef
- 3 carrots
- ½ medium rutabaga, diced
- 2 beets, chopped
- 1 T dried oregano
- 1 tsp thyme
- 1 tsp onion powder
- ½ tsp garlic powder
- ¼ tsp cinnamon
- ¼ tsp allspice
- Sea salt and pepper to taste
- 2 T tapioca flour

Directions:

I. Add everything but the flour, and cook on low for 8 hours.

II. You can use the tapioca to thicken if needed

III. Serve

Ribs and Greens

Ingredients:

- 4 lbs. bone in short ribs
- 2 T salt
- 3 C bone north
- 2 C greens

Directions:

I. Set ribs on baking sheet and season with salt and pepper and broil at 500 degrees for about 10 minutes
II. Move ribs over to slow cooker and add bone broth
III. Cook on low for around 8-10 hours
IV. Chop your greens and serve ribs over greens
V. Serve

Shredded Beef with Lemon Basil

Ingredients:
- 2 C fresh basil
- ½ C oil
- 2 T plum vinegar
- 2 T squeezed lemon juice
- 2 T minced garlic
- 3-4 lbs. beef roast
- 1/3 C bone broth

Directions:

I. Combine your first 5 ingredients in a blender or nutribullet and blend until smooth
II. Add your roaster to a slow cooker,
III. Mix your bone broth and lemon basil together, whisking to ensure blending
IV. Pour sauce over roast
V. Cook for 8 hours.
VI. Save rest of unused sauce
VII. After roasted is cooked, shred, and pour juices over shredded meat,
VIII. Add in remaining lemon sauce
IX. Serve

Pork Ribs

Pork Apple Ribs

Ingredients:

- 2 rack ribs
- 2 tsp salt and pepper to taste
- 2 tsp garlic salt
- 4 ripe apples, chopped with skin
- 1 peeled, sliced beet
- 1 medium onion, chopped
- ¼ C maple syrup
- ¼ C apple cider vinegar

Directions:

I. Add all of your seasonings and toss in a bowl or container with a lid, and toss or shake

II. Rub ribs with seasoning and cut to fit in slow cooker

III. Add everything for the rib sauce into blender and blend well

IV. Pour sauce over ribs

V. Cook on low for 6 hours for meat falling off bones, or 4 hours to eat off the bone

Roast Pork apple Gravy

Ingredients:

- 4-6 apples, peeled and cored
- 1 onion, chopped
- ¼ C water
- 5 lbs. pork roast
- 2 T EVOO
- 2 T minced garlic
- Salt and pepper to taste
- 2 tsp. thyme
- 2 tsp. rosemary

Directions:

I. Add prepared apples to the bottom of your slow cooker and add water
II. Scatter sliced onions on top of the apples, and add water (if you haven't already)
III. Add oil with rest of seasonings and rub roast
IV. Cook on low for 8-10 hours
V. When done use juices to make gravy
VI. Remove the onions, apples and juice and place into blender and mix into a gravy texture
VII. Serve

Hawaiian Pork Roast

Ingredients:
- 3 lbs. pork roast
- 6-7 C shredded pork
- 2 onion, chopped or sliced
- 3 T fresh ginger, chopped
- 1 can crushed pineapple
- ¼ C coconut water
- 2 tsp salt and pepper to taste
- 1 tsp red pepper flakes

Directions:

I.   Season your roast well and add everything into your slow cooker and cook on low for 7 hours or so.

Kahlua Roast

Ingredients:
- 5-6 lbs. butt roast
- ½ lbs. sliced bacon
- 1 ½ T Hawaiian sea salt
- 5 T minced garlic

Directions:

I.   Line your thawed bacon along the bottom of the slow cooker, and add Hawaiian salt

II.   Add your minced garlic over roast as a rub and place roast in slow cooker

III. Cook on low for 8-10 hours

Teriyaki Roast

Ingredients:
- 3 lbs. pork shoulder
- 2 T minced garlic

Teriyaki Sauce

- ¼ C Gluten free soy sauce
- 2 T fish sauce
- ¼ C organic maple syrup
- 1 ½ tsp ground ginger
- 1 T honey

Directions:

I.   Wash the pork shoulder and dry,
II.   Prepare your teriyaki sauce, with the sauce ingredients and pour into Ziploc baggie
III.   Rub roast with seasonings,   and add to Ziploc baggie, sealing for sure, and shake.
IV.   Sit in fridge overnight to marinade
V.   Add everything in to slow cooker and cook for 6-8 hours

Cantonese Ham and Root Soup

Ingredients:
- 1 ham, bone in
- 2 lotus roots, peeled, and chopped
- Red date berries
- 8-10 C water

Directions:

I.   Soak your sliced of root in the warm water, and then add to the slow cooker
II.   Add everything else remaining in the ingredients list to slow cooker and cook on low for
III. 6 hours
IV.   Remove any bones from the ham and cook another 2 hours
V.   Remove any excess bone and serve the soup (remove any added at)

Cranberry Roast

Ingredients:
- 2 lbs. pork roast
- 1 tsp salt and pepper
- 1 onion, chopped
- 3 T mince garlic
- 1 C cranberry juice
- 1 C broth
- 2 T maple syrup
- 1 T balsamic vinegar
- 2 T chopped thyme
- 1 C cranberries

Directions

I.   Season your pork and add to a skillet and cook on all sides
II.   Add your seared roast
III. Sauté your onion, garlic and remaining seasonings, then add to slow cooker as well
IV.   Pour in 2-4 C water with 2 T arrow root flour
V.   Pour juices from slow cooker into a skillet after the roast is cooked and simmer, you can add extra water or flour, whichever is needed, cook then let sit to thicken
VI.   Pour over the roast and serve

Stock Broth

Chicken Broth

Ingredients:

- Carcass from left over roasted chicken
- Any leftover chicken parts
- And 5-6 C boiling water
- 2-3 drops lemon juice

Directions:

I.   Let sit in slow cooker for 12 hours or more
II.   Strain the broth and save broth and store

Bone Broth

Ingredients:
- 4-5 lbs. beef bone marrow
- 1-2 carrots chopped
- Celery sticks, chopped
- Onion, chopped
- 4 T minced garlic
- 3 T apple cider vinegar
- Water

Directions:

I.   Sear marrow on each side briefly before adding to oven
II.   Bake for 20 minutes at 375 now add to slow cooker
III.   Cook on low for 10-12 hours , remove the bone marrow
IV.   Add veggies for 4 more hours on low
V.   Drain broth from the pot, store and save
VI.   Serve your veggies as a great side dish

Paleo Side Recipes

Crockpot Onions

Ingredients:
- 4 lbs. onions, sliced thinly
- 3 T EVOO

Directions:

I.   Peel and toss onions into slow cooker
II.   Drizzle EVOO over onions and cook on low for 12 hours
III.   Serve with steak, baked potatoes, or are on their own

Butternut Squash

Ingredients:

- Butternut Squash

Directions:

I. Get rid of the stems and slice across the long directions and get out the seeds and add to slow cooker
II. Make sure to lay the squash long directions, and add ½-1" water
III. Cook for 2 hours on high

Red cabbage

Ingredients:
- 1 red cabbage (medium to large sized)
- 2 tsp cinnamon
- ¼ C cinnamon
- 1 C cranberries
- ¼ C apple cider vinegar
- 2 large apples, cored, peeled and sliced
- 1 tsp salt

Directions:

I.   Slice your cabbage and cut out the core, and throw away
II.   Slice so your have 4 quarters and add a slit into each wedge
III.   Stir remaining ingredients in a mason jar
IV.   Add all of your sliced ingredients in to your slow cooker
V.   Cook in slow cooker for 4 hours or so
VI.   Serve

CranApple Sauce

Ingredient:

- 15 apples cored, and peeled
- 1 C fresh cranberries
- ½ tsp ginger
- ½ lemon juice
- ¾ C raw maple syrup
- 1 tsp pure vanilla
- ½ tsp raw cinnamon
- ¼ C water
- Salt to taste

Directions:

I.   Add everything into your slow cooker
II.   Set on low and cook for 4-5 hours, you want apples to be very tender, falling apart
III.   Turn slow cooker off, break down apples, and serve warm

Apple Butternut Curry Soup

Ingredients:
- 2 lbs. coconut oil
- 2 C chopped onions
- 1 T turmeric powder
- 1 T ground ginger
- 2 lbs. butternut squash, cubed
- ½ lbs. apples, cored and peeled, and chopped
- 5 C bone broth
- 1 tsp Himalayan salt
- Green apples

Directions:
- Heat oil up in skillet and sauté your onions, add seasoning, for 5-6 minutes or so on low
- Add everything to your slow cooker and cook on low for 6 hours
- Puree in blender and serve

Printed in Great Britain
by Amazon.co.uk, Ltd.,
Marston Gate.